Epilepsy

A patient handbook

Dr Jim Morrow

BA (Hons), MD, PhD, FRCP

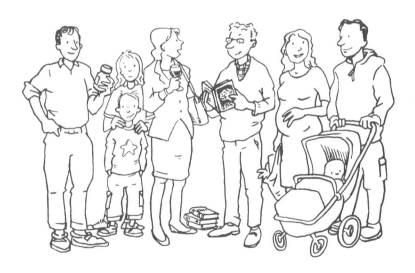

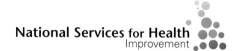

National Services **for Health**
Improvement

Epilepsy: A Patient Handbook
by Dr J Morrow

Published in the UK by:

National Services for Health Improvement

Nucleus@The Bridge

London Science and Business Park

Brunel Way, Dartford DA1 5GA

Copyright 2010 NSHI Ltd.

Printed in the UK by Stephens & George Print Group

ISBN 978-0-9560921-7-5

About the author

Dr Jim Morrow is a Consultant Neurologist at the Royal Group of Hospitals, Belfast and also an Honorary Reader with Queen's University, Belfast. Previously he was a Clinical Lecturer in the University Hospital of Wales where he was involved with the early clinical trials of many of the newer anti-epileptic drugs that are now firmly established in day to day clinical practice. His postgraduate Doctorate thesis examined the physical, social and occupational handicaps associated with epilepsy and in particular the benefits of specialised epilepsy clinics in the clinical management of patients with epilepsy.

Within Northern Ireland he has established a number of dedicated, specialist epilepsy clinics and in conjunction with a team of specialist epilepsy nurses he now additionally provides a pre-conceptual service for women with epilepsy and a joint Obstetric/Epilepsy clinic. He is lead clinician in Neurology and co-ordinates the Northern Ireland Epilepsy Service, and also acts as a Specialist Advisor for Epilepsy Action in Northern Ireland and the United Kingdom.

Jim has published widely on these and many other related subjects in the field of epilepsy. He has participated in National Guidelines committees on the treatment of refractory epilepsies, the UK Guidelines group on the management of women with epilepsy and the Royal Society of Medicine's Primary Care Guidelines group on the management of females with epilepsy. He is the founder and principal investigator of the UK Epilepsy and Pregnancy Register, a nationwide register that monitors the outcomes of pregnancies in women with epilepsy, with particular reference to the potential teratogenic effects of the anti-epileptic drugs.

Contents

Introduction

Despite being such a common condition, it is often surprising how little people actually know and understand about epilepsy. It is not that long ago that epilepsy was a taboo subject, often hidden from others and still, I suppose, most people don't feel the need or perhaps don't want to know about the condition, yet epilepsy can affect anyone; it does not discriminate.

Perhaps the reason that you have picked up this booklet is because you, a relative, or a friend has had a seizure and you want to understand more about the condition. Maybe you want to know what it is, why you or your friend or relative has got it, how it is diagnosed and treated, what it will mean to your/their lifestyle and what will be the outcome.

Jimi Hendrix once said 'Knowledge speaks, but wisdom listens'. This booklet sets out to try to 'speak' to you to explain the condition, its implications and its treatment in an easy to read format and I hope that you can 'listen' to it and learn something from it.

I hope that this booklet will help to dispel many of the myths associated with the condition and help you realise that even though the diagnosis may come as a shock at first, epilepsy is usually easily treatable and life should carry on much as before.

I hope you find it useful.

Jim Morrow
April 2010

Chapter 1

What is epilepsy and what type do I have?

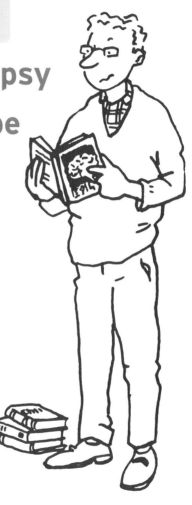

What is epilepsy and what type do I have?

Seizures are no respecter of age, sex, class or culture; anyone can have an epileptic seizure at anytime in their life. A seizure is what happens when there is a sudden abnormal burst of intense electrical activity in the brain. The brain functions normally on electrical activity (something that can be measured during an EEG test) but a seizure occurs when this intense burst of activity causes a disruption of the normal working of the brain.

An epileptic seizure is the manifestation of this electrical burst and may come in many shapes or forms. For example, it may manifest itself simply as a sensation or feeling that only the person themself is aware of, or it may take the form of a short period of unawareness or blankness which the person themself may not be totally aware of, but which those around them may notice, or it may take the form of a full blown tonic clonic ('convulsive' or 'grand mal') seizure. What a person experiences depends on where and over what area of the brain this burst of intense electrical activity occurs.

Doctors try to sub-divide or classify epilepsy and individual seizures as this helps them plan further investigations, helps them choose the best treatment and gives them an idea of the likely future outcome (the prognosis), i.e. chances of the seizures stopping.

Seizures can start at any age; however, most commonly they start in early childhood or in later life. In childhood epilepsy, there is usually not a cause, but in epilepsy starting in the middle years of life or more commonly in later years of life, there is often an underlying cause.

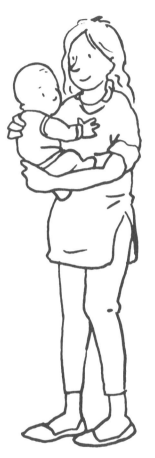

Types of seizures

Doctors try to determine what type or types of seizures are occurring in an individual patient. They do this almost exclusively from the history or description of the seizures given to them by the person who has the seizure and/or by an eye witness account from someone who has witnessed the seizure or seizures occurring.

Doctors divide seizures into partial (or focal) seizures, secondary generalised seizures, and primary generalized seizures.

Partial (or focal) seizures are those which, as the name implies, involve an intense burst of epileptic activity occurring intermittently but in just one part of the brain. The effect that this produces will depend on the area of the brain in which the activity occurs. Partial seizures are generally sub-divided into what is termed 'simple partial' and 'complex partial' seizures. By simple partial seizures it is meant that the person involved remains conscious throughout the attack. In a complex partial seizure the patient loses awareness of their environment to a greater or lesser extent.

Secondarily generalised seizures are those which start as a partial seizure (in one part of the brain) but then spread to the rest of the brain, usually then resulting in a tonic clonic (grand mal or convulsive) seizure. The partial (or focal) onset may be determined by the symptoms that the person experienced prior to going into the major seizure; however, this partial onset may be very rapid or may be forgotten after the seizure is over, so that it can be difficult to distinguish primary generalised tonic clonic seizures (see below) from those with a partial (or focal) onset.

Primary generalised seizures are those in which the abnormal electrical activity appears to start over the whole surface of the brain simultaneously. Primary generalised seizures can come in a number of different forms. The commonest types are absences seizures, myoclonic seizures and tonic clonic seizures; tonic seizures and atonic seizures are less frequently seen.

Individual seizure types

Partial seizures

Partial seizures arise when the abnormal electrical activity occurs in one area of the brain. This can happen in any area but is probably most commonly linked with the temporal lobes of the brain.

Partial seizures may arise as a result of some small scarring in one area of the brain which can result from a previous injury or infection (the temporal lobes are particularly prone to injury or infection). But any injury or infection may even have occurred prior to birth and therefore not be remembered by patient or relative. Such scars, however, may be of such small size that even modern day scans will not necessarily detect them.

Simple partial seizures

A simply partial seizure is a seizure which comes from one area of the brain. It usually does not spread very far and gives rise most commonly to sensations of which the person is fully aware. The effected person remains conscious throughout the seizure. Common sensations include an intense déjà vu feeling ('I've been here before'), a feeling of something rising up from the stomach or a feeling of fear or anxiety. Another common sensation usually attributed to seizures from the temperal lobe is a sensation of taste or smell, though other sensations may occur in individuals, depending on the site of the epileptic activity. When the seizure does not progress but remains simply as a sensation, it is often referred to as an aura.

Usually, in any individual, the sensation that occurs is the same every time. It will usually come on suddenly, for no apparent reason, and will last only for matter of seconds and then pass. However, because the person who experiences this type of seizure remains fully aware of what is happening throughout, they often find these sensations quite upsetting or distressing.

Another type of simple partial seizure not infrequently seen is a simple motor seizure (sometimes called a 'Jacksonion seizure' after the doctor who first described it). In this is a type of seizure, because the epileptic activity is occurring in the motor cortex of the brain, i.e. the area that controls the movement of the limbs, rather than it producing a sensation, there is rhythmical shaking of a limb. Characteristically, the shaking or twitching starts in the hand or the foot but may progress to involve the whole of the limb or the whole side of the body, though the affected person remains fully conscious of this movement. On occasion, this localised activity may spread to become a full blown secondarily generalised tonic clonic seizure. Sometimes, focal seizures coming from in and around the motor cortex may be followed by a period of temporary paralysis of the arm and or leg after the seizure is over. Such paralysis can last for minutes to hours but usually resolves completely and is known as a Todd's paralysis.

Complex partial seizures

A complex partial seizure is a seizure which is occurring in one part of the brain but it is distinguished from simple partial seizures in that the person loses awareness of their surroundings, i.e. they cannot interact with individuals around them; they may look as if they are aware and alert but they are not able to respond normally to those around them. Often when the seizure has abated they can't remember the seizure afterwards and they may be confused for a short period of time following it.

A complex partial seizure may follow on from a simple partial onset, i.e. the person may experience some of the sensations described above before they lose awareness of their surroundings; however, this does not always occur and many patients go straight into a complex partial seizure.

In a complex partial seizure the person involved is not usually aware of what is happening and it is at this point that the eye witness account is of great value. An eye witnesses may describe the person staring or looking blankly and often going a bit pale. They may describe what are termed automatisms. These are short periods of automatic behaviour. Typical automatisms include lip smacking or chewing mouth movements, fumbling with buttons or items of clothing, the head turning to one side as if looking around at something, or sometimes arms and legs moving in strange and complicated ways. The person may even get up and walk around whilst still unaware of their surroundings. As this short period of seizure activity wanes, these automatic behaviours will cease, the person will become more aware of their surroundings but may be somewhat confused for a period of time afterwards.

Secondarily generalised seizures

Any of the above seizures, whether simple or complex partial, may progress if the electrical activity spreads across the brain to a secondarily generalised tonic clonic seizure. The major seizure will therefore be preceded by some of the symptoms described above. However, such spread may be very rapid and indeed in many cases almost instantaneous, so that it is sometimes difficult to determine whether a tonic clonic seizure is a primary generalised tonic clonic seizure (see below) or a secondarily generalised event.

Primary generalised seizures

Absences

Absence seizures are probably the commonest type of primary generalised seizures and are usually seen in childhood. They only occur infrequently in adults, as many children who develop them grow out of them as time goes by.

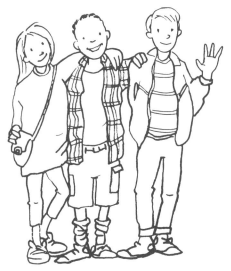

These seizures are often of a very minor nature in that it may appear to observers that the child is simply daydreaming. They usually just stop what they are doing, may stare blankly and perhaps blink a little. The event is very short lived (a few seconds) and then they resume where they left off. The child is usually totally unaware that anything has happened. Often, however, these episodes occur very frequently, i.e. many times per day, and as a result may lead to a fall off in school performance due to the constant inter-ruptions to concentration. School teachers are often very good at picking up these minor seizures.

Complex partial seizures are often mistaken for absences, but can be distinguished if there is an 'aura', 'automatisms' and/or after effects (such as a period of confusion), which are uncommon with absences.

Myoclonic seizures

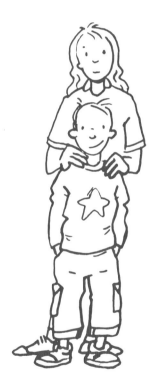

The most common type of myoclonic seizures occur in the form of epilepsy termed 'juvenile myoclonic epilepsy'. This type of epilepsy tends to present in the teenage years. It usually starts with some intermittent jerks of the limbs, particularly the arms. These happen most often in the morning, usually if the affected person has not slept well or has been woken early in the morning. In later years they may also be precipitated by alcohol. These jerks may be associated with absence seizures, i.e. short periods of staring and blinking, but because of their fleeting and minor nature they are often ignored. Sometimes the jerks can be severe enough to cause the dropping of objects, particularly in the morning and usually over breakfast, hence this type of epilepsy is often referred to as 'cornflake epilepsy', 'teacup epilepsy' or even 'flying saucer epilepsy'.

If the significance of these myoclonic jerks is not recognised then it is very likely that a generalised tonic clonic seizure will eventually occur. Once again, this usually happens in the morning time and then in retrospect the history of these short lived jerks will give away the seizure and epilepsy type that is occurring.

Tonic clonic seizures

Tonic clonic seizures (convulsive or grand mal seizures) are most people's perception of what an epileptic seizure actually is, though as this book hopes to demonstrate, there are many different seizure types, most of which are of a much more minor nature.

Typically, in a tonic clonic seizure the affected person will go unconscious and collapse to the ground. They may give a cry, their body will stiffen and then this is followed by convulsive

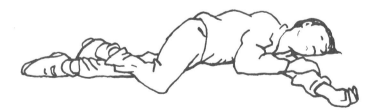

movements of the limbs. Seizures will usually terminate after a few minutes but the affected person may be very drowsy or confused for a period of time afterwards. They may find that their tongue or cheek has been bitten during the seizure and they may have involuntarily passed urine.

Tonic clonic seizures can be either primarily or secondarily generalized, depending if the electrical activity starts in one area or occurs over the whole brain surface at the outset.

Tonic seizures

In these seizures the person affected goes stiff and falls to the ground "like a tree trunk" without any convulsive activity.

Atonic seizures

In atonic seizures the person suddenly loses their muscle tone and falls limply to the ground. It is in these seizures and in tonic seizures that injury is most likely to occur, as they are sudden events with no warning, which invariably result in falls.

Types of epilepsy

Epilepsy is defined as a tendency to recurrent seizures. Doctors tend to group epilepsies by their cause. There are three groups. These are idiopathic, cryptogenic and symptomatic.

Idiopathic epilepsy
Idiopathic epilepsy is where there is no apparent cause for the seizures.

Cryptogenic epilepsy

Cryptogenic epilepsy is a type of epilepsy where the doctors believe that there is an underlying cause but they have not been able to find it.

Symptomatic epilepsies

Symptomatic epilepsies are those for which a cause for the seizures has been found.

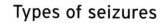

What is epilepsy and what type do I have?

Types of seizures

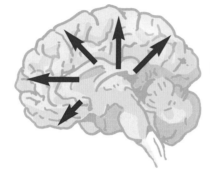

Generalised

Idiopathic
Symptomatic
Cryptogenic

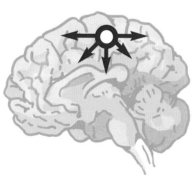

Focal/Partial

Chapter 2

How do doctors diagnose epilepsy?

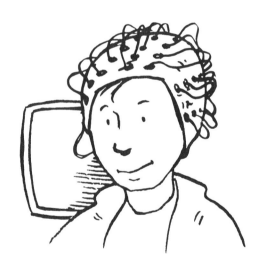

How do doctors diagnose epilepsy?

Epilepsy is defined as a tendency to recurrent epileptic seizures; therefore a diagnosis of epilepsy will rarely be based on a single event. Seizures themselves may come in many different shapes and forms and these have been described in the previous chapter.

Contrary to popular opinion, there is no test for epilepsy, although tests can be helpful in guiding and informing the doctor in working toward the correct diagnosis and in initiating treatment.

The most important aspect in making a diagnosis of epilepsy from the doctor's stand point is the description (or history) of the event or events that have been occurring. While sometimes the person who experiences the seizures may be partially or even fully aware of the events themselves, it is usually important to have someone who has seen one or more of the episodes accompany the affected person to the initial consultation with the doctor. This is very useful to the doctor, as seizures often involve an impairment or loss of consciousness or awareness, and this eye witness will be able to fill in the history of the attacks during the time that the person who experiences them is not fully aware.

The most important aspects of the history of the attacks are:

- **What happened before the attack?**
- **What happened during the attack?**
- **What happened after the attack?**

What happened prior to the attack?

It is important to be aware of the circumstances in which the attack happened. In particular, are there any triggers or precipitating factors that may have provoked it?

Also, any symptoms that preceded the attack may be important. There are some symptoms that commonly precede seizures but

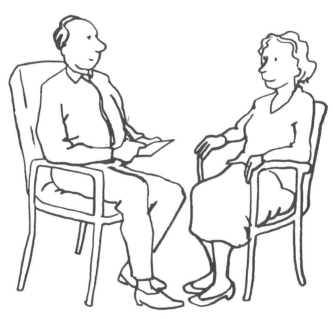

there may be other symptoms which would be unusually associated with seizures and may suggest an alternative cause, for example, chest pain or palpitations (which might suggest a cardiac cause). Perhaps the most common events that get confused with epilepsy are fainting attacks (syncope). The symptoms that precede the blackout are often helpful in distinguishing the true nature of the event(s), e.g. a feeling of blackness descending over the affected person, or things fading away, are generally more suggestive of a faint than a of a seizure.

Symptoms that suggest a warning of an epileptic seizure (or aura) would include:

- **A feeling of déjà vu ("I've been here before")**
- **A feeling of jamais vu ("I've never been here before")**
- **A smell or taste sensation**
- **A feeling of apprehension**
- **A feeling of something rising up from the stomach and spreading over the head**

There are of course many other sensations or feelings that may herald a seizure and these can be particular to the individual. Usually though, auras are stereotyped, that is it is usually the same sensation each time it occurs.

What happened during the event?

Sometimes peoples will remain fully conscious during the event and be able to describe what is happening to them during the attack, but very often consciousness is impaired or lost during the seizure itself and usually, therefore, an eyewitness may be of most value in filling in the gaps as they can describe to the doctor what was occurring during the actual attack.

◆ **Did the person fall to the ground?**

◆ **Did they appear to remain conscious?**

◆ **Did they respond to questioning?**

◆ **Was there any unusual behaviour or movement?**

◆ **Was there any stiffening or shaking of the limbs?**

◆ **How long did this period of unconsciousness last?**

If an eye witness cannot come to the appointment with the doctor, then discussing the above questions with them, or bringing their written account, may help the doctor to come to a diagnosis.

What happened after the event?

Sometimes the person themselves may be able to recall how they felt immediately after the attack.

◆ **Did they come round quickly?**

◆ **Were they confused and sleepy for a while?**

◆ **Had they fallen or injured themselves?**

◆ **Had they bitten their tongue or their cheek?**

◆ **Had they passed water during the event?**

An eye witness account may, however, again be of value, particularly if a person has been somewhat confused for a period of time following the event.

The most common alternative explanation for a blackout or blackouts occurring in a young person is fainting attacks (syncope). *Table 1* highlights some of the similarities and differences in the symptoms that may occur before, during and after a syncopal attack as opposed a seizure.

Table 1: Some of the characteristic features that MAY occur in fainting attacks and/or epileptic seizures.

Possible features	Seizure	Faint
Warning	Yes/no	Yes
Pallor	No	Yes
Seizure activity	Yes	No
Tongue biting	Yes	No
Incontinence	Yes	No
Rapid recovery	No	Yes

It should, however, be noted that none of these symptoms are completely or mutually exclusive of each condition. For example, a warning may occur before a syncopal attack or before an epileptic seizure but these warnings may be different. Before a syncopal attack it may be a feeling of things fading away or blackness coming over a person, whereas the warning for an epileptic attack may be a more typical epileptic aura, a feeling of déjà vu, a strange smell or taste, or a feeling of something rising up from the stomach.

In syncopal attacks, typically people will go pale but this can occur in some epileptic seizures as well; it is not uncommon in partial onset seizures for example. Shaking or twitching of the limbs is most commonly associated with a tonic clonic (grand mal) type seizure. However, such activity can also occur in fainting attacks, particularly if the person who faints does not collapse completely flat on the ground. When one faints, the pulse and blood pressure drop, so the brain is essentially starved of oxygen supply and reacts by causing the person to fall flat so that the blood supply is restored. However, if the person for some reason remains in a partially upright position, for instance if they are caught and held up by someone else or if they fall into a chair or against a wall so that they don't become completely flat, then some seizure activity with shaking of the limbs may occur but is of non serious import and does not necessarily imply that an epileptic seizure has happened – seizure activity of this sort, as part of a faint, is often called a reflex anoxic seizure. In contrast, in many types of epileptic seizures there is no such overt seizure activity. In absence seizures or in minor partial seizures, the patient may simply switch off and not be totally aware of the surroundings but there may be no frank epileptic activity.

Tongue biting is most commonly associated with tonic clonic type seizures but does not necessarily occur and usually does not happen in minor epileptic events. It can occur in faints if, for example, one falls and hits the ground so that the tongue gets trapped between the teeth in the fall.

Incontinence of urine is most commonly associated with an epileptic seizure but may occur in fainting episodes; for example, if the person has got out of bed quickly to go to the toilet because their bladder is full and then faints, it would not be surprising if they had a degree of incontinence.

After seizures, one usually associates a slow recovery with some period of confusion or drowsiness but after some seizures, e.g. absence seizures, people recover completely almost immediately. After fainting attacks a quick recovery is usual but if a person has fallen and hit their head they may be dazed and confused for a time afterwards.

In summary, no individual or single symptom should be given undue weight in making the diagnosis of a seizure or a faint but, rather it is the entire picture surrounding the event or events that needs to be considered and it is this that a doctor will usually do in trying to come to a diagnosis.

Most doctors who treat epilepsy will take the diagnosis very seriously. This is because the diagnosis itself carries with it a number of significant issues. Usually it will bring with it the need to take regular and long term medication. It will bring with it a number of possible social, occupational and economic consequences. In particular, a person who is subject to epileptic seizures would not be considered eligible to drive a motor vehicle until they can demonstrate at least 12 months of seizure freedom. This clearly can have an impact on a person's social and occupational wellbeing. Many employed people encounter difficulty with their employers once a diagnosis of epilepsy is made, particularly if their job involves working at heights or with moving machinery.

If doctors are uncertain whether what have been described to them are epileptic seizures, they may take the view that it is best not to treat until certainty is obtained. However, it is prudent to take precautions in case further blackouts or seizures might occur; for example, it may be important to refrain from driving until a diagnosis is reached, whether it be epilepsy or not. Bathing may be considered dangerous and showering is preferred. If one goes swimming, it may be advisable at least for a period of time to be accompanied by a responsible adult so that no mishaps occur.

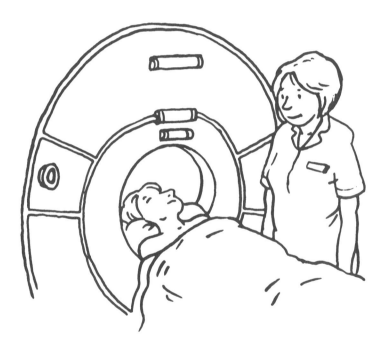

Investigations

When a doctor has taken the history and completed an examination in order to try to reach a diagnosis, they may consider some investigations to aid in this diagnosis. Usually a GP who suspects epilepsy will refer the patient to a specialist at a hospital, usually a paediatrician or a neurologist. The specialist may order a number of tests to help reach a firm diagnosis. These include:

1. Blood tests
A doctor may take blood tests to check on overall health and to rule out any underlying medical condition that may be responsible for the blackouts.

2. An EEG (electroencephalogram)
An EEG is a harmless investigation which records the electrical activity in the brain. It involves placing electrodes on the scalp and doing a recording of the normal electrical activity of the brain. It may be possible during this investigation to pick up some abnormal or epileptic type discharges, even though no frank seizure activity is detected. However, it should be noted that in the majority of patients, the EEG between attacks proves to be normal and is therefore non-conclusive.

3. Prolonged video EEG (VEEG) monitoring
On occasion, particularly if a person is having frequent repeated episodes, it may be possible to admit the patient to hospital for a few days to carry out a prolonged VEEG test. This involves placing the person in a room with a video camera and an EEG attached to the person continuously over a number of days in the hope of picking up epileptic activity. If epileptic

activity is picked up through either the standard EEG or the prolonged EEG, then this may help guide the doctor, not only in diagnosing that the attacks are due to epilepsy but also the type of epilepsy or seizure that is occurring, which in turn may help in the selection of the correct drug therapy.

4. CT scan (computerised tomography)

This scan is a type of detailed x-ray which looks for any areas of abnormality or damage in the brain that could be giving rise to seizures.

5. MRI scan (magnetic resonance imaging)

An MRI scan does not involve x-rays but produces pictures of the brain by using high powered magnets. These scans are more sensitive to small lesion such as small scars within the brain, which may again give rise to seizures.

6. Other tests

A number of other tests including SPECT (single photon emission computerised tomography), PET (positron emission tomography) or Depth EEG electrodes (electrodes inside the skull itself) may be carried out in specialised centres where seizures prove to be frequent and resistant to anti-epileptic drug therapy; such tests are not usually carried out unless drug therapy has failed.

Chapter 3

Are there things I should avoid?

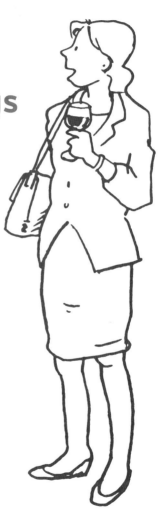

Are there things I should avoid?

The question "are there things I should avoid?" encompasses two separate subjects. The first group of things to avoid are what are termed 'precipitants', i.e. things or situations that may provoke seizures, and the second group of circumstances or situations to avoid are those in which a person may become injured if a seizure were to occur.

Precipitants

There are certain things or situations that may precipitate epileptic seizures in those prone to seizures. However, every person is different, and while some people may be sensitive to certain things, others may not. The following list discusses a few of the more commonly recognised precipitants of epileptic seizures.

Flickering lights

Rapidly flickering lights such as may be encountered in a disco, a flickering television screen or a video or computer game, or even by sunlight flickering through railings or trees, are a recognised precipitant of epileptic seizures in some people. However, this association has been greatly over emphasised. In actual fact, less than 5% of people with epilepsy have seizures which can be triggered by flashing or flickering lights. The type of epilepsy that is triggered by this type of stimulus is called 'Photo Sensitive Epilepsy' and can often be detected during an EEG test. Photo sensitivity is most common with the idiopathic primary generalised epilepsies *(see chapter 1)*.

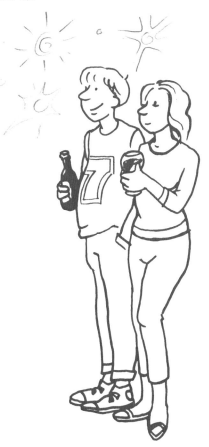

If you are a person who is photosensitive, even then not all flickering or flashing lights will provoke an epileptic seizure. It is usually only flickering or flashing lights at a certain frequency (usually between 12-24 flashes per second) that may cause you a problem. Closing one or both eyes, turning away or quickly leaving the area if such flickering occurs, will usually prevent any attack from happening.

Photosensitive seizures usually happen at the time of, and in front of, the flickering or flashing lights; they do not usually occur sometime afterwards.

Alcohol

Alcohol is a recognised precipitant of epileptic seizures and is perhaps one of the commonest causes of seizures seen in the United

Kingdom. Seizures related to alcohol usually occur the morning or the day after alcohol intake.

It is even recognised that seizures may be provoked in people who do not have epilepsy if they partake in heavy alcohol binges. In such cases, the treatment is usually not the prescription of anti-epileptic drugs but rather a modification of lifestyle.

Recreational drugs

Most recreational drugs have been associated with the provocation or precipitation of epileptic seizures. Some people believe that cannabis may provide protection against epileptic seizures but because it is taken intermittently, as it wears off it may in fact precipitate seizures, and therefore the general advice is to avoid recreational drugs if one has epilepsy.

Prescription drugs

Some prescription medications may lower the seizure threshold and result in seizure breakthrough by a direct effect on the brain or by interfering with the anti-epileptic drugs. The most common drugs that are associated with this problem are anti-depressant drugs. Most recently it has become apparent that the commonly prescribed anti-epileptic drug, lamotrigine, may have its effect lessened by the addition of the oral contraceptive pill, which could result in seizure breakthrough. However, your doctor should know about these interactions and should discuss these with you before prescribing additional medications if you are taking anti-epileptic drugs.

Herbal and complementary medications

There is evidence that some herbal or complementary medications may precipitate seizures and are best avoided:

◆ **Evening Primrose Oil has been noted to cause seizures in people with some focal epilepsies**

◆ **St John's Wort may interfere with the effect of some of the anti-epileptic drugs**

◆ **The aromatherapy oil containing Rosemary has been reported to lower the seizure threshold**

As with most herbal or complementary medicines, these remedies are not exposed to the rigorous testing that prescription medicines are; therefore one should always treat them with a certain amount of caution and it is worth discussing them with your GP or neurologist.

Fatigue and tiredness

It is generally recognised that fatigue, tiredness and lack of sleep can precipitate seizures in those prone to them and should therefore be avoided if at all possible.

Concomitant illness

Concomitant illness or stress, whether physical or emotional, may precipitate seizures. Clearly such stressors are difficult to avoid but an awareness of their effect on seizure frequency should be noted.

Travel

Travel per se, including air travel, does not usually precipitate epileptic seizures. However, tiredness, dehydration and alcohol consumption, which may occur during travel, may have effects on the likelihood of seizures.

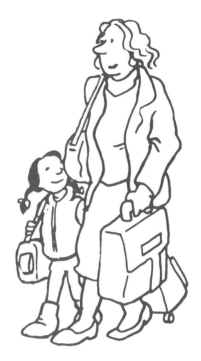

It is always important, however, when travelling to take an adequate supply of medication in your hand luggage as it is not uncommon for luggage to be lost and the acute cessation of anti-epileptic medication may in itself precipitate epileptic seizures.

What should I do to avoid injury?

Clearly the answer to this question depends on the nature and frequency of any epileptic seizures that are occurring and can only therefore be answered in individual cases taking into account these factors. Some general points, however, may be made.

Driving

Anyone subject to periods of altered or loss of consciousness (whether due to seizures or some other cause) should not drive a motor vehicle and indeed are generally legally barred from doing so. It should be noted that in the UK it is the person's own responsibility to report any such events to the DVLA.

The dangers are obvious. Even a momentary lapse in concentration may result in a road traffic accident, with potentially serious consequences.

In general terms, the legal requirement for driving following a diagnosis of epilepsy is that the person must demonstrate a period of 12 months of seizure freedom and be on stable medication before being legally allowed to drive a motor vehicle.

Cycling

If you have poorly controlled epilepsy it is best to avoid busy or public roads and it is recommended that you always wear a helmet when cycling (good advice whether you have epilepsy or not!)

Bathing

It is generally recommended that because seizures can be unpredictable, and even if very infrequent, that showering is preferable and safer than bathing.

People with epilepsy can often obtain a grant to have a shower put into their house if one is not already present.

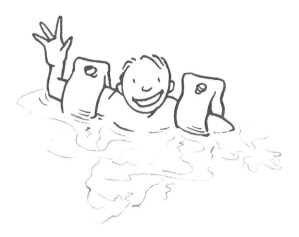

Swimming

If seizure free or if seizures are well controlled, there is generally little risk if you swim in a pool that is supervised by a qualified lifeguard or you take a friend or relative with you. Always tell the life guard that your have epilepsy.

Swimming when the pool is quiet is generally a good idea and you should not swim if you feel unwell or feel that you are likely to have a seizure. Swimming in a river or sea can be dangerous; however, once again having a relative or friend with you who is aware of your condition may lessen the risk.

Heights

Again, any advice should be on an individual basis but if seizures are frequent or unpredictable, then working at heights, such as up a ladder, on a roof or climbing, may place you in a situation of undue risk and should be avoided at least until the epilepsy is controlled.

Contact sports

In general terms, epilepsy should not be a bar to playing football or rugby, but if your epilepsy has been caused by head injury you should discuss with your doctor any contact sport that you wish to play.

Boxing is a sport that most doctors will advise to avoid because there is a risk of being hit on the head and it is recognised that blows to the head may precipitate or cause seizures.

Going to the gym

If seizures are well controlled there is usually no problem using any piece of gym equipment. It is probably best though to take advice from one of the instructors at your gym, who should be able to advise you as to which pieces of equipment in particular would be safe to use, avoiding injury to yourself or others should a seizure occur.

Fishing or water sports

It is usually advisable when fishing or partaking in other water sports, such as sailing, to have someone with you who is aware of your condition. This is particularly important if your seizures are frequent or unpredictable. The wearing of a life jacket is another important (and simple) measure to help avoid injury.

When fishing it is usually safer to fish from a riverbank, rather than a boat or pier.

Scuba diving

Scuba diving is not usually recommended and can be quite dangerous if you have epilepsy. If you have a seizure while scuba diving it could prove fatal. Anti-epileptic medication may also heighten other risks of scuba diving such as disorientation. The UK Sport Diving Medical Committee recommends that someone with epilepsy should only scuba dive after they have demonstrated five years seizure free, without taking anti-epileptic medication.

Other sports

It is probably wise to get your doctor's approval before you take part in other sports, particularly extreme sports such as parachuting, bungee jumping, paragliding etc. Some of these sports have safety regulations with a governing body, which may put restrictions on people with epilepsy. It is always worth checking.

Chapter **4**

Should I
start treatment?

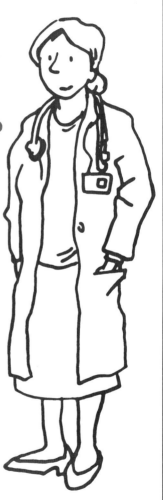

Should I start treatment?

The question of whether to and when to start treatment is an individual decision, and should be made in careful consultation with your doctor.

In general terms, doctors will not usually recommend starting treatment after a single epileptic seizure, but will if seizures are recurrent. Once treatment is initiated, for all practical purposes a diagnosis of epilepsy has been established and this may carry with it, not only the necessity to continue on treatment in the longer term, but may also impose some social and occupational handicaps. Therefore, the diagnosis of epilepsy is never taken lightly.

A single seizure

A single epileptic seizure does not constitute epilepsy and many people will have a seizure but never go on to have any more. It must be recognised, however, that after a single unprovoked epileptic seizure, there is a definite risk of further seizures occurring. Studies in this area suggest that the chance of a second or more seizures occurring within the next 12 months, following the initial event, may be around 50-60%. This risk is highest in the early months and then falls off fairly quickly, so that if seizures are going to recur, it is usually sooner rather than later.

If there has been a single epileptic event which has no obvious provoking or other cause, usually doctors will not advise anti-epileptic drug therapy, but instead will advise taking precautions in case of any further events, i.e. not driving, bathing, swimming etc.

If, on reviewing the history of the event, it transpires that there has been something which has provoked the seizure, then the treatment in any case may not be with drug therapy, but rather simply to avoid the provoking factor in the future.

As with any rule, however, there are of course exceptions about not treating single events. After a single epileptic seizure, if an underlying cause for the seizure has been found and this cause is still present, for example an abnormality on a scan or if an EEG is carried out and reveals ongoing epileptic activity, even without any obvious seizure activity, then the doctor may feel that the risk of further clinical seizures breaking through is very high and therefore drug therapy may be recommended even at this early stage.

Recurrent seizures

If a person has recurrent, i.e. more than one, epileptic seizures then they are usually considered to have 'epilepsy', at which point it is usually advisable to start treatment to prevent further seizures from occurring. However, it is generally considered good medical practice not to prescribe anti-epileptic drug therapy until a diagnosis is secure. A 'trial of drug therapy' is usually doomed to failure. Trials of drug therapy may result in patients being prescribed anti-epileptic medication with the wrong drug or at the wrong dose because the doctor is unclear about the seizure type, or just wrongly because the blackouts are not due to epilepsy at all. In other words, if the events are not witnessed or they are not felt to be typical of epilepsy, it is usually best not to start anti-epileptic treatment until there is more clarification about the true nature of the events. Of course, because there is a risk of further events during this time, precautions should be taken to avoid accidents or injury.

If it becomes clear that the diagnosis is one of epilepsy and this diagnosis is secure, then it usual to start anti-epileptic drug therapy as early as after the second seizure. The selection of drug therapy will depend on a choice between the predicted efficacy of the drug (i.e. how well the drug will work against the particular seizure type), balanced against the risk for any side effects of that drug in that individual person.

The initiation and choice of drug therapy is therefore usually best carried out by a specialist in the field of epilepsy, and your GP should refer you for confirmation of the diagnosis and advice regarding starting drug therapy.

Once again, as with any rule, the rule that drug therapy is started after the demonstration of recurrent seizures has its exceptions. For example, on occasions a seizure may occur and there may actually have been one previous event, but the earlier event was many years ago. In such cases there is an argument to be made to start therapy, but as the risk of more seizures, at least in the short term, is probably low, there is also a case not to start therapy unless there was an escalation of attacks. Other examples might be cited and in these cases it is advisable to have the opportunity to discuss them in detail with your specialist, who will be able to help you weigh up the pros and cons of starting drug therapy.

If the seizures are clearly 'provoked', for example following alcoholic binges, then the treatment may be an alteration in lifestyle rather than medication. In such cases, medication may actually worsen the situation by providing a false sense of security and if medication is omitted or forgotten whilst drinking, the withdrawal from the medication may actually make it more likely that a seizure will happen.

As in many areas of medicine, it is often a matter of patient choice. Some patients or parents of patients may be very resistant to drug therapy. However, if events are recurrent, there is a real risk of even further events occurring. It needs to be appreciated that seizures do carry inherent dangers, particularly where and when they occur, and therefore lifestyle issues and potential areas of risk need to be fully discussed with the specialist.

If drug therapy is agreed and prescribed, then the importance of taking the medication regularly cannot be over emphasised. If drug doses are missed, particularly if they are missed recurrently, then there is a high risk of seizure breakthrough, and sudden or abrupt cessation of drug therapy can actually cause epileptic seizures. Therefore, a commitment has to be made at the outset of treatment to try to take the medication on a regular and ongoing basis. Once a commitment to anti-epileptic drug therapy is made it is usually recommended that it is continued until one can demonstrate a prolonged period of seizure freedom. This is usually in the order of a minimum period of some 12-24 months.

In most cases, anti-epileptic drug therapy is very effective and one generally expects about 60-70% of people to become seizure free once drug therapy is initiated. The vast majority of these will become seizure free, often on low doses of the first drug prescribed. In some, however, drug therapy may need to be altered, either because of side effects of the first drug or because it proves ineffective against the seizures. In such cases, a second drug may be introduced and the first drug withdrawn. Unfortunately, in a significant minority of patients, seizures may continue despite initial drug therapy. If seizures continue, it is certainly worthwhile asking your GP about referral (or re-referral) to an epilepsy specialist, as further options do exist.

These options include:

- **Review of the diagnosis**
- **Combinations of drug therapy (polytherapy)**
- **Use of the newer anti-epileptic drugs that have been emerging over the last 10 years**
- **Surgical options for treatment of epilepsy**

All of these options are discussed more fully in *Chapter 5*.

Chapter 5

What treatment is best for me?

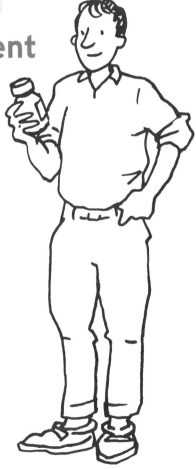

What treatment is best for me?

The main way of treating epilepsy is with anti-epileptic medication. Once the correct drug and the correct dosage have been found, for most people the seizures should cease.

Prescriptions for anti-epileptic medication are free and to claim you should obtain form FP92A from a hospital chemist or your doctor.

Anti-epileptic drugs usually come in tablet form but if you have difficulty swallowing tablets then for many of the drugs there is a syrup or soluble form available.

When started on anti-epileptic medication it is important that roughly the same amount of the drug stays in the bloodstream day and night. Missing doses or taking a medication much later than normal can lower the drug level in the blood and this can lead to seizures. Too much medication can also cause side effects and occasionally may also lead to an increase in seizures.

Which drug is best for me?

Different anti-epileptic drugs act on the brain in different ways to prevent seizures. Some drugs are better for certain types of epilepsy than others and your doctor will give you advice about the best drug for you. There are a number of factors that your doctor will take into consideration; these are:

◆ **The type of epilepsy that you have**

◆ **Your age**

◆ **Whether you are male or female**

◆ **Your medical history**

◆ **Other drugs that your are taking**

◆ **Your lifestyle**

What is the correct dosage?

In general terms, the correct dosage is the lowest dose that stops the seizures. It is usually advisable to start on any anti-epileptic drug at a low dosage and then to increase it slowly. All too often these drugs are started at too high a dose or too quickly and then side effects result. The aim is to achieve seizure control on the lowest amount of the drug possible. This will minimise the risk of any side effects.

It should be noted that everybody may react differently to drugs, so there is a degree of trial and error in trying to find the right drug and the right dose for any individual. If the seizures continue or there are side effects, the doctor may elect to change the dose or even the drug itself. It will be helpful to the doctor if you record your seizures in a diary and make a note of any adverse effects that occur between visits.

Below is a list of the commonly used anti-epileptic drugs with the type of seizures that they are most often used to control and possible side effects that have been associated with each drug. It should be noted that side effects are possible with any drug but usually do not occur in the majority of people.

Anti-epileptic drugs always have two names: a 'generic name' and a 'brand name'. The generic name is the chemical name of the drug and the brand name is the name given to the drug by the manufacturer who first makes it. The brand name is usually copyrighted by that manufacturer. After a drug has been around for a period of time, other manufacturers are allowed to produce the drug. They are not, however, allowed to use the brand name. 'Generic prescribing' (i.e. prescribing by the generic name, so that the drug can be sourced from a number of manufacturers) is now common place, as alternative manufacturers can often produce drugs much cheaper than the original manufacturer of the branded drug. It is noteworthy, however, that generic formulations made by a number of manufacturers are not necessarily identical to the original drug or each other, and small variations are allowed to persist. In the majority of people these small differences will have no effect, but in certain individual cases may result in changes in the blood level of the anti-epileptic drug, which in turn may result in seizure breakthrough or toxic effects. While these changes may be small, the results, particularly if there is seizure breakthrough, can have disastrous consequences upon driving, work and social life. In many cases, therefore, it is advisable to insist that your doctor writes the brand name and not the generic name on your drug prescription to try to ensure that you get the same drug each time you go for a repeat prescription.

Table 2: Anti-epileptic drugs prescribed for various seizure types, and possible side effects

Name Generic/Brand: **Carbamazepine/Tegretol**

Seizure type: Partial seizures or generalised tonic clonic seizures (NB - may worsen absence or myoclonic seizures)

Possible side effects: Skin rash, sedation, blurred or double vision, unsteadiness, drowsiness

Name Generic/Brand: **Clobazam/Frisium**

Seizure type: Tonic clonic seizures, myoclonic seizures and partial seizures

Possible side effects: Drowsiness, dizziness, blurred vision

Name Generic/Brand: **Clonazepam/Rivotril**

Seizure type: Tonic clonic seizures, myoclonic seizures and partial seizures

Possible side effects: Drowsiness, sedation, dizziness

Name Generic/Brand: **Ethosuximide/Zarontin**

Seizure type: Absence seizures

Possible side effects: Skin rash, drowsiness, headache, nausea, vomiting, irritability, dizziness

Name Generic/Brand: **Eslicarbazepine acetate/Zebinix**

Seizure type: Partial seizures with or without secondary generalisation

Possible side effects: Dizziness somnolence, headache, tremor, blurred vision

Name Generic/Brand: **Gabapentin/Neurontin**

Seizure type: Partial or secondary generalised seizures

Possible side effects: Drowsiness, dizziness, blurred vision, weight gain

Name Generic/Brand: **Lacosamide/Vimpat**

Seizure type: Partial seizures with or without secondary generalisation

Possible side effects: Dizziness, unsteadiness, double vision, drowsiness, nausea, vomiting

Table 2: Anti-epileptic drugs prescribed for various seizure types, and possible side effects (continued)

Name Generic/Brand: Lamotrigine/Lamictal

Seizure type: Partial secondary generalised absence, myoclonic and tonic clonic seizures
(NB - in some cases may worsen myoclonic seizures)

Possible side effects: Skin rash, nausea, double vision, dizziness, insomnia

Name Generic/Brand: Levetiracetam/Keppra

Seizure type: Partial seizures and generalised seizures

Possible side effects: Drowsiness, mood change

Name Generic/Brand: Oxcarbazepine/Trileptal

Seizure type: Partial and secondary generalised seizures

Possible side effects: Skin rash, double vision, unsteadiness, nausea, confusion

Name Generic/Brand: Phenobarbitone/Primidone/Mysoline

Seizure type: Tonic clonic seizures, myoclonic seizures, partial seizures

Possible side effects: Drowsiness, sedation, mental slowing, behavioural problems in children

Name Generic/Brand: Phenytoin/Epanutin

Seizure type: Tonic clonic, partial seizures and generalised tonic clonic seizures

Possible side effects: Skin rash, drowsiness, unsteadiness, slurred speech, over growth of the gums, acne-like symptoms

Name Generic/Brand: Piracetam/Nootropil

Seizure type: Myoclonic seizures

Possible side effects: Skin rash, dizziness, insomnia, nausea, diarrhea, weight gain, mood change, drowsiness

Name Generic/Brand: Pregabalin/Lyrica

Seizure type: Partial seizures and secondary generalised seizures

Possible side effects: Dizziness, drowsiness, blurred or double vision, mood change, weight gain, concentration difficulties

Table 2: Anti-epileptic drugs prescribed for various seizure types, and possible side effects (continued)

Name Generic/Brand: Rufinamide/Inovelon

Seizure type: Seizures associated with Lennox-Gastaut Syndrome

Possible side effects: rash, nausea, vomiting, abdominal pain, weight loss, dizziness, tiredness

Name Generic/Brand: Sodium valproate/Epilim

Seizure type: Partial seizures and generalised seizures

Possible side effects: Nausea, vomiting, hair loss, weight gain, tremor, irregular menstrual cycle

Name Generic/Brand: Tiagabine/Gabitril

Seizure type: Partial and secondary generalised seizures

Possible side effects: Dizziness, fatigue, drowsiness, diarrhoea, headache, mood change, confusion

Name Generic/Brand: Topiramate/Topamax

Seizure type: Partial seizures and generalised seizures

Possible side effects: Tiredness, drowsiness, mental slowing, speech arrest, weight loss, pins and needles in the hands and feet, tremor

Name Generic/Brand: Vigabatrin/Sabril

Seizure type: Partial and secondary generalised seizures

Possible side effects: Drowsiness, fatigue, weight gain, mood change, confusion (NB - may cause visual field loss)

Name Generic/Brand: Zonisamide/Zonegran

Seizure type: Partial seizures with or without secondary generalisation

Possible side effects: Dizziness, drowsiness, nausea, diarrhoea, weight loss and confusion

What if the treatment doesn't work?

The vast majority (60-70%) of people with epilepsy will have complete seizure freedom on anti-epileptic drug therapy. However, there will remain some who continue to take seizures. In the majority of these, however, the drug therapy will usually lessen the severity and the frequency of the seizures, so that while there is not a complete effect from the drugs, there is at least a partial effect.

Therefore, in some 30-40% of people, seizures do continue. This may be because there are underlying abnormalities which make the epilepsy more resistant to treatment than in other cases. In some cases it may be due to ongoing lifestyle issues such as irregular sleeping patterns, binge drinking etc, which may continue to precipitate epileptic seizures and these may need to be addressed. If seizures continue, however, it is usually worthwhile seeking the opinion of an Epilepsy Specialist, as nowadays there are a wide range of medications and other therapies that may be available which may not have been considered. It is worth talking to a GP about onward referral to an epilepsy specialist if adequate seizure control is not achieved. An epilepsy specialist will usually start at the beginning, as one of the common causes for ongoing events is that the person may not actually have epilepsy at all. There are a number of alternative diagnoses that may superficially sound or look like epileptic seizures but, in fact, are not epilepsy. An epilepsy specialist will usually go over the history of the events from the patient and from an eye witness, very carefully, to ensure that the diagnosis is correct. They will also review the medication because not all medications work for every type of epilepsy or every individual, and there may be an issue regarding alternative medications.

Certainly, the last 10-20 years has seen an upsurge in the number of anti-epileptic drugs available, and the number of the newer drugs may offer more in individual cases than the older or more conventional anti-epileptic drug therapies. An epilepsy specialist would be best placed to consider this. Further investigations may be helpful in delineating the diagnoses and/or type of epilepsy to aid the specialist to review the diagnosis. One of the investigations would be VEEG, whereby prolonged EEG recordings can be taken to record the events that are occurring to firstly ensure that they are definitely epileptic and, secondly, to classify the type of seizure and epilepsy that is occurring, which may further guide treatment.

MRI scanning may be repeated in a Specialist Centre to try to delineate underlying structural or other abnormalities that may be giving rise to the ongoing epileptic seizures. In some cases, the events turn out to be non-epileptic but may instead be related to cardiac or syncopal (fainting) issues, which may need to be addressed by a Cardiologist. In other cases, the seizures may turn out to have a psychological basis, and sometimes psychological or disassociated seizures may occur along with true epileptic seizures. Seizures which are not truly epileptic do not respond to anti-epileptic drug therapy but may respond to other forms of therapy, such as psychology input etc. One should always keep an open mind regarding these possibilities. For true ongoing epileptic seizures, a number of surgical options may be considered. One of the commonest causes of ongoing epileptic seizures is scarring in the temporal lobe (hippocampal sclerosis); this can be delineated on an MRI and the epileptic discharges can sometimes be picked up on prolonged EEG recordings.

In these cases the removal of the scarred area (temporal lobectomy) may result in complete seizure freedom and ultimately withdrawal of anti-epileptic drug therapy. However, this is only possible if there is a single epileptic focus and it can be found. Other surgical options tend to be reserved for much more refractory cases and tend to be much less successful than a temporal lobectomy. Vagal Nerve Stimulation is a less evasive surgical intervention, in which electrodes are placed on the vagus nerve in the neck and connected to a pacemaker type device inserted in the chest. The pacemaker, via the electrodes, stimulates the vagal nerve on a regular basis and this has been shown to reduce, but rarely abolish, the severity and frequency of epileptic seizures and may be useful as an adjunct therapy to traditional medical therapy. All of these options would be considered by an epilepsy specialist.

Are there other treatments apart from drugs?

For the vast majority of people with epilepsy, anti-epileptic drug therapy is the treatment of choice and is usually very successful. There are a number of alternate therapies but these are mostly used in conjunction with anti-epileptic medication, at least initially, and usually are not considered unless seizures continue despite anti-epileptic medication.

These therapies include:

Ketogenic diet

This is a diet which has been available for many years. It has been shown to be helpful in reducing seizure frequency and severity in children with epilepsy that has proven very difficult to control with medication. Essentially, it is a diet which involves increasing the fat content in the diet. It should only be tried under medical supervision. It is often felt to be a somewhat unpleasant and a generally unhealthy diet to take in the longer term. It has not, to date, been shown to be effective in adults and even in children who respond to it, it is rarely sufficient by itself to stop seizures.

Complementary alternative therapies

Complementary medicines are becoming increasingly popular with patients who may use them in addition to conventional medication. However, there is no evidence to support the use of acupuncture, herbal medicines, osteopathy or yoga in place of conventional anti-epileptic drug therapy. There is some evidence however, to suggest that aromatherapy may aid

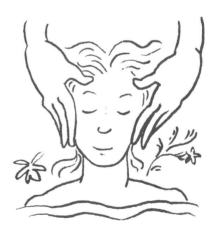

seizure reduction in combination with anti-epileptic drug therapy. Whether this works simply through relaxation techniques or through the effects of the oils used, is uncertain. The epilepsy societies, however, suggest that some aromatherapy preparations are best avoided. These include rosemary, hyssop, sweet fennel, sage and wormwood.

It should be noted that some herbal medications may interact with prescribed anti-epileptic drugs, reducing their concentration and thus possibly resulting in seizure breakthrough. St John's Wort, for example, may reduce the serum concentration of carbamazepine, phenobarbitone and phenytoin. There have been some other reports linking oil of evening primrose and ginkgo biloba, to seizure provocation.

Surgical treatments

Surgical treatments for epilepsy are generally only considered when drug therapy (usually after a number of drugs have been tried) has failed. An exception to this rule may be when scans have revealed an underlying (and accessible) cause for the seizures. In such cases a neurosurgical referral may result in the removal of the underlying abnormality and hence, possible cessation of the seizures. Even in such cases, the temporary use of anti-epileptic medication may be required.

In cases where epilepsy has proven to be resistant to anti-epileptic drug therapy, other surgical interventions may be considered.

These include:

Temporal lobectomy

By far the most successful surgical intervention for people with
proven refractory (i.e. difficult to
control epilepsy) is temporal
lobectomy. In this form of surgery part of the temporal lobe is
removed. This is successful in
controlling epilepsy only if it has
been demonstrated through a
variety of detailed investigations
that the epilepsy is arising within that area of the temporal lobe
and that further investigations
have revealed that it would be
safe to remove this area of the
temporal lobe without damage
to the individual involved. Such
surgery is usually carried out in
specialised centres but, if possible, is highly successful.

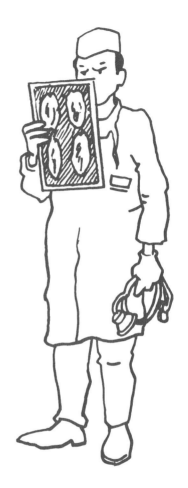

Corpus callosotomy

This is a surgical procedure in which there is a partial splitting of
the corpus callosum (this normally acts like a bridge between the
left and right halves of the brain). This surgery is only usually car-

ried out in children with very resistant epilepsy. By splitting the corpus callosum, any seizure activity cannot spread across the brain from one side to the other, i.e. seizures cannot generalise. This operation therefore does not usually stop seizures completely but may reduce their severity by limiting the area of the brain involved. Because this separation of the right and left parts of the brain may have other effects on normal functioning, it is generally only considered in very resistant cases.

Vagal nerve stimulation (VNS)

Vagal nerve stimulation is a less invasive form of surgery than the above two examples. It involves putting a small pacemaker type device under the skin in the chest wall and connecting it via electrodes to the vagal nerve in the neck. This pacemaker device then stimulates the vagal nerve regularly at intervals. This stimulation has been shown to reduce seizure frequency and severity in some patients with previously difficult to control epilepsy. Only in a very small percentage of patients does it ever abolish seizures completely, and most people need to continue on anti-epileptic drug therapy.

Chapter 6

What if I want to have children?

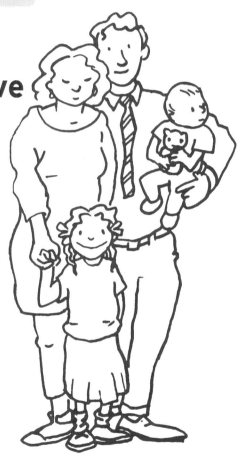

What if I want to have children?

Deciding whether or not to have a baby is a major decision for many women, but especially so for those women who have epilepsy. A number of thoughts may come to mind:

◆ **Will the anti-epileptic drugs or the seizures affect my unborn child?**

◆ **Will it be safe for me to look after my baby?**

◆ **Will the baby inherit my epilepsy?**

These are perhaps just a few of the questions that are in potential mothers' minds. Because there are recognised risks in association with epilepsy and the anti-epileptic drugs during and after any pregnancy, it is important to plan ahead so that the decisions about the drugs and/or the control of epilepsy can be made before the pregnancy occurs.

Contraception

Contraception is an issue in planning for pregnancy and there are many contraceptive options available. Some anti-epileptic medications, those termed enzyme inducing drugs, may interfere with the oral contraceptive pill and make it less effective. These drugs include carbamazepine, phenytoin, topiramate (at higher dosage), phenobarbitone, primidone and oxycarbazepine. If you are taking one of these drugs then, because the ordinary dose of the oral contraceptive pill may be ineffective, it is usually advisable for your GP to increase the dose of the oral contraceptive, but even then contraception cannot be guaranteed and it is advisable to use a barrier method of contraception as well as the pill.

If you are someone who is taking lamotrigine, it is important to be aware that whilst the contraceptive pill may work normally, the level of lamotrigine may fall when the pill is started and this increases the risk of seizures.

Other methods of contraception such as Depo-Provera, the intrauterine device (coil), are generally not affected by (nor effect) any of the anti-epileptic drugs.

Pre-conceptual planning

If you are planning a family it is important to seek pre-conceptual counselling. This may be from your GP, but most GPs will refer you on to a specialist to discuss the issues in more detail.

It should be borne in mind that the vast majority (more than 90%) of women with epilepsy will have completely healthy babies, whether they are taking anti-epileptic medication or not.

It is important to ensure that your health is as good as possible before becoming pregnant.

Some women may wish to try to reduce or even to stop their medication prior to pregnancy. It would be important to discuss this with a specialist prior to doing so. Abrupt or sudden cessation of anti-epileptic drug therapy can be very dangerous indeed, resulting in increased seizure activity and even status epilepticus (a series of uncontrolled seizures). Any reduction or withdrawal of medication should be slow, gradual and planned.

It will take time to reduce or withdraw anti-epileptic medication successfully, once a decision is made to do so, and as it may take many months to withdraw or reduce medication, there is a need to plan well in advance.

For many women with epilepsy, it may be inadvisable to reduce or withdraw medication because the risk of seizures is too high. In which case, recent studies are suggesting that some drugs carry less risk to the baby than others. It should be emphasised however, even for those drugs in the higher risk category, the absolute risk remains low, with more than 90% of children born to women taking these drugs, being healthy and well. Once again, your specialist or epilepsy nurse may be able to advise whether a change in drug therapy would be worthwhile considering prior to any pregnancy.

The UK Epilepsy and Pregnancy Register phone line (Free Phone 0800 389 1248) is available to answer any questions or queries that you may have and may be able to put you in touch with your local Specialist Epilepsy Service.

Folic acid

Folic acid is a vitamin which has been shown to protect babies from developing neural tube defects (spina-bifida). When planning a family it is generally recommended that women with epilepsy take 5mg of folic acid every day (this is higher than the standard 0.4 mg dose usually given to pregnant women). It should be taken for at least three months before you conceive and continued throughout the pregnancy, if possible. This strength of tablet is only available on prescription and your GP will know if it is suitable for you.

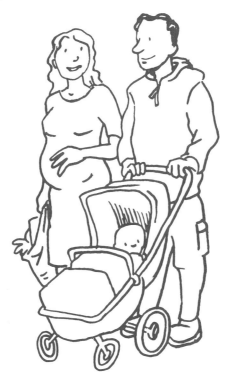

During pregnancy

Many women experience no change to seizure frequency during pregnancy and some notice an improvement. However, for about a third of women the frequency of seizures may increase. This may be due to reduced levels of the drugs in the bloodstream, perhaps due to sickness, changing effects of hormones, increasing blood volume as the baby develops, or increased metabolism and clearance of the drugs from the body. Your doctor will monitor your condition and sometimes it may be necessary to increase your medication to keep you healthy and maintain seizure control during the later stages of pregnancy and labour.

Generally speaking, unborn babies are rarely harmed by the mother having a seizure, unless the mother falls and injures herself. Tonic clonic (grand mal) seizures are obviously more of a risk than the other more minor seizure types. Status epilepticus (a series of uncontrolled seizures) is rare, but can cause harm to the mother and the unborn child. It is therefore important to try to maintain seizure control during pregnancy.

In general terms the best advice is to try to control the epilepsy as well as possible with the lowest amount of medication as possible.

Vitamin K

Vitamin K helps to maintain the clotting factors in the blood. Most babies routinely receive vitamin K when born and sometimes the mother is prescribed oral vitamin K in the last month of pregnancy as it is thought to be beneficial in counteracting a very rare complication called "hemorrhagic disease of the newborn". It is thought that if a woman is taking one of the enzyme inducing anti-epileptic drugs (carbamazepine, phenytoin, topiramate, phenobarbitone, primidone or oxcarbazepine), taking 20mg of vitamin K daily in the last month of pregnancy may be useful in this regard. It is not generally recommended for any of the other medications. Once again, this tablet is only available on prescription.

Coping with labour

Providing you and your baby are well, the epilepsy should not prevent you from having a normal labour or delivery. You will generally be advised to have your baby in hospital to minimise the risk of any complications that may arise. You should always remind doctors and midwives that you do have epilepsy and it may be useful to ask your midwife or your birth partner to remind you to take your medication, at the usual times during labour. As many obstetric units do not always have a supply of anti-epileptic drugs, it is useful to pack your medication in the bag that you intend to take with you to hospital.

TENS machines, gas and air and epidurals can all be used for pain relief. Pethidine, however, is thought to have a convulsant effect and therefore should be avoided if at all possible.

Scans and tests during pregnancy

There are a number of tests, such as scans and blood tests, avail- able for all pregnant women. Some of these tests check on the baby's development and look for abnormalities in the child. These tests are particularly helpful if it is considered that your baby has a higher risk of a birth defect due to your epilepsy or the anti- epileptic drugs. This is something you should discuss with your obstetrician, who can then plan which scans and tests to do and when to do them during your pregnancy.

Post-pregnancy

Breastfeeding

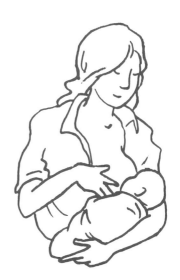

Breastfeeding is generally recommended for all babies. A small amount of the anti-epileptic drug will pass to the baby in the breast milk; this usually has very little or no effect on the baby. Sometimes people are advised not to breastfeed because some of the older anti-epileptic drugs could cause excessive sleepiness in the baby, but this is now rare with the newer anti-epileptic drugs more commonly used today. It would be important to discuss the benefits and risks of breastfeeding with your specialist and your specialist epilepsy nurse.

Bear in mind that if you do breastfeed, your nighttime sleep will be broken on a regular basis and if lack of sleep is a known trigger for your seizures, this is a factor which may need consideration.

Caring for children

Most people with epilepsy successfully care for babies and young children. However, if your seizures are not well controlled then there are some precautions that you may wish to take to make sure that your baby is as safe as possible. These include:

◆ Try not to become too tired or exhausted as this may trigger seizures

◆ When feeding a baby from a bottle or your breast, you should sit on the floor, on a towel or a rug, so that if you had a seizure, your baby does not fall

◆ Never bath a baby or child on your own; instead give them a simple sponge bath or seek support from another adult

◆ Change a baby's nappy on the floor; changing units are not usually recommended as the baby could roll off if you had a seizure

◆ When carrying a baby up and down stairs, use a car seat to provide protection from a fall

◆ Use a pram with a brake which comes on when you release the handle

◆ When you take a child out, use reins that are attached to you and them to prevent the child wondering off if you became unconscious

◆ Teach a child as soon as possible what to do if you have a seizure; children are remarkably adaptable

◆ As with all medicines, make sure all your anti-epileptic drugs are locked away from children at all times

Inheriting epilepsy

Many parents worry that their children might inherit their epilepsy. Whilst it is true that children who have a parent with epilepsy do have a slightly higher risk of developing it, overall this risk is actually quite small. Less than one child in every ten born to a parent with epilepsy will themselves go on to develop epilepsy.

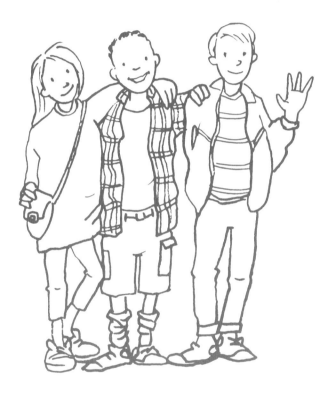

There are three main ways in which epilepsy can be inherited:

◆ **A person's low epileptic seizure threshold may be passed onto the next generation through their genes**

◆ **Some types of epilepsy seem more likely to run in families**

◆ **Epilepsy can be one of the symptoms of another inherited medical condition, e.g. tuberous sclerosis**

If you are worried that your child might be at risk of inheriting epilepsy, or if you have a family history of epilepsy, it would be worth talking to your GP or epilepsy specialist and they may decide to refer you on to a Genetic Counsellor who will try to work out with you the risk of your child developing epilepsy.

Chapter 7

Can I come off treatment?

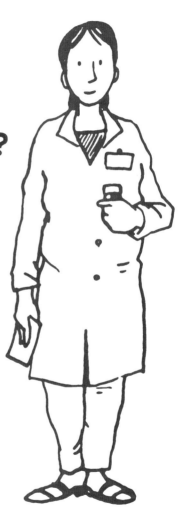

Can I come off treatment?

The question of stopping treatment usually arises in one of two circumstances:

◆ **There have been no seizures for some time**

◆ **Seizures are continuing and there is a question over whether the treatment is effective**

Seizure freedom

The majority of people who develop epilepsy will eventually become seizure free (over 60%), usually with a single anti-epileptic drug, though some people will require more than one drug to achieve seizure freedom. Many people who become seizure free grow out of the propensity to seizures and may therefore successfully withdraw from drug therapy. This is true for probably up to two-thirds of people who become seizure free on drugs. However, once seizure freedom is obtained, it is important to maintain it over a period of time before considering drug withdrawal.

Drug withdrawal should never be embarked upon lightly and should always be considered very carefully. In general terms it is considered wise to discuss the pros and cons, and the risks and benefits of drug withdrawal with an epilepsy specialist before starting to alter a successful dosage regime.

A recurrence of seizures is more likely if:

◆ **There is an underlying cause for the epilepsy which has not gone away**

◆ **The epilepsy was difficult to control at the outset**

◆ **There are certain seizures types, e.g. myoclonic seizures**

It is for these reasons that the former history of the epilepsy, the response to therapy, and results of previous investigations, need to be carefully considered before embarking on drug withdrawal and these are probably best assessed by an epilepsy specialist.

Unfortunately, there is no test that will predict the outcome or success of drug withdrawal, an EEG test for example, if carried out before drug withdrawal is likely to prove to be normal but is this because the epilepsy is controlled by the drugs or because it has gone away? The only true 'test' of whether seizures will recur is to start a slow drug withdrawal and keep aware of the possibility of seizure recurrence. It cannot be overemphasised that there is always a real risk of seizure recurrence and that this may have social and occupational consequences, which need to be carefully considered in each individual case prior to attempting drug withdrawal.

In general terms, doctors tend to be more proactive in attempting drug withdrawal in the cases of children and teenagers, as the consequences of a further seizure are usually less than for an adult in whom a recurrence of seizures will result in the loss of a driving licence and other difficulties.

The consequences on driving, in particular, deserve special consideration. As anyone thinking about drug withdrawal will usually be seizure free, and eligibility to drive depends on seizure freedom (in the UK one is eligible to drive after 12 months clear of seizures). Many people will therefore be driving at the time they are considering drug withdrawal. Because there is a risk of seizure breakthrough and because the timing of any seizure is unpredictable, there is a general recommendation that driving should be suspended whilst drug withdrawal is taking place and for up to six months after the drug is withdrawn, as these are considered the times of greatest risk of seizure recurrence. Drug withdrawal, therefore, involves a prolonged period of not driving, even if no seizures occur (and longer if seizure recurrence does occur). The effect that this may have on lifestyle needs careful consideration prior to attempting drug withdrawal. Because of these issues, it may be important to consider the prospect of drug withdrawal in the teenage years before driving becomes an issue.

Generally, doctors will not usually recommend drug withdrawal unless a patient has demonstrated a prolonged period of seizure freedom. For children this is usually in excess of one year and for adults it is usually in excess of two years. On occasion or under special circumstances, earlier drug withdrawal may be considered.

If a drug or drugs are to be withdrawn then a graduated regime should be drawn up and in general terms it is considered good practice to withdraw drugs one at a time and to withdraw each individual drug over a minimum period of approximately three months. The greatest risk of seizure recurrence is during the withdrawal phase and within the first few months thereafter.

If one is continuing to take anti-epileptic medication it may be difficult to make an argument that one doesn't have epilepsy any more, even if there have been no seizures for quite a long time. One advantage of drug withdrawal, if successful, is that one can certainly be considered as not having epilepsy any more, and this may be beneficial from a psychological, social and occupational point of view.

Drug withdrawal with continuing seizures

In some cases, seizures continue despite anti-epileptic drug therapy and many people in this situation may question whether the drugs are working at all, and therefore whether there is a need to continue. This should be discussed in every individual case, preferably with an epilepsy specialist.

Although drug therapy may superficially seem not to be effective, it may in fact be providing some level of control of the seizures whilst not abolishing them completely. The drug may, for example, be limiting the severity or the duration of seizures but this may not be obvious to the individual involved. The risk of status epilepticus, i.e. continuous or recurrent seizures, is always present and can be potentially very dangerous. The risk of status epilepticus is reduced by taking anti-epileptic medication, even if the drug therapy does not appear to be controlling individual seizures.

It is increasingly recognised that seizures are potentially dangerous and can even prove fatal. This is principally because of where they occur. If a seizure were to occur at the wrong time or in the wrong place, for example up a ladder, driving a car or having a bath, then this clearly places the individual at considerable risk. It should also be noted that seizures per se can be fatal, giving rise to a condition termed SUDEP (Sudden Unexpected Death in EPilepsy). This is a situation in which a seizure occurs and there is an associated cardio-respiratory arrest, which may result in sudden death. Although this is rare, it is increasingly recognised and is a risk that is related to inadequate control of seizures.

If it is perceived that seizures are not being controlled by an individual anti-epileptic drug, this should be discussed preferably with an epilepsy specialist. It may be that the wrong drug or the wrong dosage is being used for the particular seizure or epilepsy type, and that adjustment needs to be made. These adjustments may be either in dosage or therapy. When change is required it is usual for a second drug to be added before a subsequent withdrawal of the first drug that appeared ineffective.

Appendix 1: First aid for epilepsy

If you have a friend or a relative who has epilepsy, or if you witness an epileptic seizure, the following is a general guide of what to do in the event of such a seizure.

DO

- TRY TO GUIDE OR PROTECT THE PERSON FROM INJURY, I.E. REMOVE HARMFUL OBJECTS FROM NEARBY

- IF THEY ARE LYING ON THE GROUND, CUSHION THEIR HEAD

- LOOK FOR AN EPILEPSY IDENTITY CARD OR IDENTITY JEWELLERY

- IF THE PERSON IS HAVING A MAJOR SEIZURE, AID BREATHING BY GENTLY PLACING THE PERSON IN THE RECOVERY POSITION ONCE THE IMMEDIATE SEIZURE HAS FINISHED

- STAY WITH THEM AND BE CALMING AND REASSURING

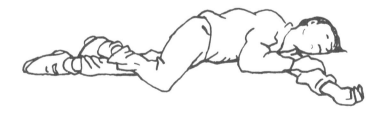

DON'T

- TRY TO RESTRAIN THE PERSON
- PUT ANYTHING IN THEIR MOUTH
- TRY TO MOVE THEM UNLESS THEY ARE IN DANGER
- GIVE THE PERSON ANYTHING TO EAT OR DRINK UNTIL THEY ARE FULLY RECOVERED
- ATTEMPT TO BRING THEM ROUND

CALL AN AMBULANCE

CALL AN AMBULANCE IF:

- YOU KNOW IT IS A PERSON'S FIRST SEIZURE
- THE SEIZURE CONTINUES FOR MORE THAN FIVE MINUTES
- ONE TONIC CLONIC SEIZURE FOLLOWS ANOTHER WITHOUT THE PERSON REGAINING CONSCIOUSNESS BETWEEN THE SEIZURES
- THE PERSON HAS INJURED THEMSELVES DURING THE SEIZURE OR YOU BELIEVE THE PERSON NEEDS URGENT MEDICAL ATTENTION

Appendix 2: Sources of further information

Epilepsy Action (British Epilepsy Association)
New Anstey House, Gate Way Drive, Yeadon, Leeds LS19 7XY

Tel: 0113 210 8800
Helpline: 0808 800 5050
E-mail: helpline@epilepsy.org.uk
Website: www.epilepsy.org.uk

The National Society for Epilepsy
Chesham Lane, Chalfont St Peter, Buckinghamshire SL9 0RJ

Tel: 01494 601300
Helpline: 01494 601400
Website: www.epilepsynse.org.uk

Professional website: www.e-epilepsy.org.uk
website for individuals with a professional interest in epilepsy; the
information is relevant to GPs and they can e-mail questions directly
to the medical experts at NSE.

The National Centre for Young People with Epilepsy
St Piers Lane, Lingfield, Surrey RH7 6PW

Tel: 01342 832 243
Helpline: 01342 831342.
E-mail: info@ncype.org.uk
Website: www.ncype.org.uk

Epilepsy Scotland
48 Govan Road, Glasgow G51 1JL

Tel: 0141 427 4911
Helpline: 0808 800 2200
E-mail: enquiries@epilepsyscotland.org.uk
Website: www.epilepsyscotland.org.uk

UK Epilepsy and Pregnancy Register
c/o Dr JI Morrow, Department of Neurology,
Royal Victoria Hospital, Grosvenor Road, Belfast BT12 6BA

Helpline: 0800 389 1248
Website: www.epilepsyandpregnancy.co.uk

DVLA
Swansea SA99 1BN

Tel: 0870 240 0009 (general enquiries);
0870 600 0301 (medical adviser)
Website: www.dvla.gov.uk

Epilepsy Bereaved
PO Box 112, Wantage, Oxon OX12 8XT

Tel: 01235 772850
Bereavement contact line: 01235 772852
Website: www.sudep.org

This organisation does not offer a counselling service, but is pleased to help and support bereaved relatives through its bereavement contact line above.

Index

Notes

Notes

Notes